Essential Oils For Beginners:

Easy Guide To Get Started With Essential Oils And Aromatherapy

Table of Content :

Essential Oils For Beginners:

Best Guide To Get Started With Aromatherapy
and Organic Recipes With Essential Oils

Ella Witt

Essential Oils For Beginners

Best Guide To Get Started With Aromatherapy and Organic Recipes With Essential Oils

Introduction

Since the ancient times it is known that essential oils are very beneficial to our overall health. Before we experienced the advancement of modern medicine, essential oils are already present because they are already been used by our forefathers in several purposes.

When it comes to ingredients you will not find any flaws on them because they are completely all-natural or in other words they are a product of different herbs that are combined together to become worthy of your attention.

Before I was really skeptical about it because I thought how come will an essential oil cure such ailments? I tried several ways on how to cure my asthma but did not find any answer even on the medicines that the doctor is giving me that's why, what I did is to go for alternative medicines. This is where I came across the so-called essential oils, I did not knew that it will take a lot of effect on my overall health in a positive way.

To tell you frankly, my problem with my asthma has been completely resolved. I was really shocked with the results because I did not expect that a natural way of healing will suffice the need to cure my chronic condition.

Within a few days, my chronic condition got healed which made me feel happy because I felt a lot of relief. This is the primary reason why I decided to create a book that tackles the different essential oils that you can utilize to help you with your dilemmas.

I personally tried these recipes and they are really effective that's why you are in good hands because you have the peace of mind that it will work and you do not need to experiment anymore because I experimented them and tried it myself.

So by imparting these recipes with you, I have this joy of sharing and at the same time helping you to become overall well. Do not worry because all of the essential oils that we will tackle here are completely safe to use. And as a matter of fact I did not experience any allergic reactions from them.

As you will notice in the following chapters there are essential oils that are repeated because they have more than one use. It is the fact because herbal medicines are proven to target more than one condition.

Do not worry because it does not mean that if you are using an essential oil it tells that you have sickness because essential oils can be used for various purposes which we will discuss further in this book. So brace yourselves as we dive deeper into the different essential oils and their corresponding uses.

Chapter 1 – Essential Oil Recipes For Stress and Anxiety

Stress is prevalent nowadays and became a part of our day to day existence here on the planet. It is an immediate action of our body to combat the threats that we have either negative or not. The dilemma happens when stress stays longer than usual, which results in depression and other types of mental illnesses.

The Role of Essential Oils in Relieving Stress

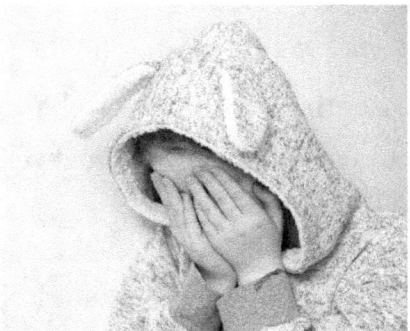

Stress can originate from different scenarios that we experience in our lives. We are lucky that there are natural techniques to support you in recovering from stress so that it will not elevate into something worse.

Thankfully, the concept of essential oils is invented because of them a lot of problems can now be cured naturally without any hassles.

They are very effective in releasing stress aside from that they can also enhance our performance and energy on everything that we do. Scientific research with essential oils particularly citrus has shown a significant improvement in their mental state.

Here are some examples of essential oil recipes that you can do at the comforts of your own home to relieve stress without undergoing any medical procedure.

Lavender and Clary Sage Blend

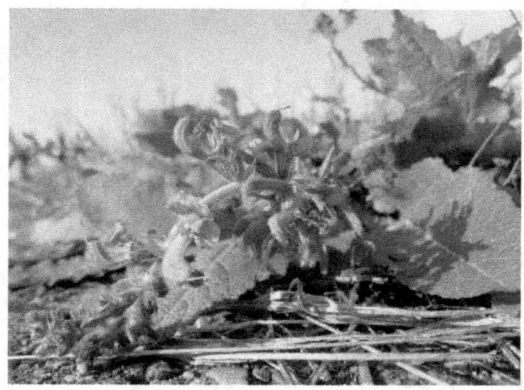

There are instances that stress can lead to sleep deprivation. The proceeding combinations of essential oils will aid you in sleeping rapidly which will result in lessening of stress in your life.

Lemon oil (5 drops)

Clary Sage (8 drops)

Lavender oil (5 drops)

Almond oil (2 drops)

Massage the combination of those essential oils among your hands and breathe in the aroma. Then continue doing it at the back of your neck and downwards. You can sense the pressure being released out of your body.

Sandal Wood Essential Oil Blend Recipe

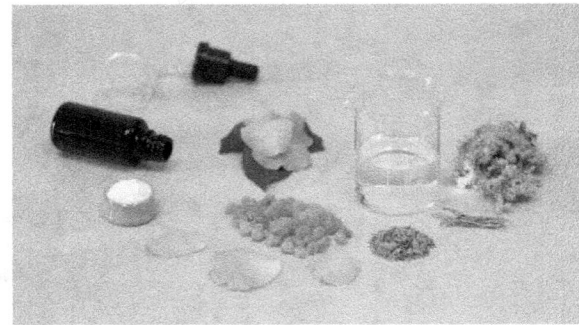

Put 5 drops of vetiver and 5 drops of sandalwood to the water that you will be used in taking a bath and then unwind while gasping the aroma.

Ylang-Ylang and Valerian Essential Oil Blend Recipe

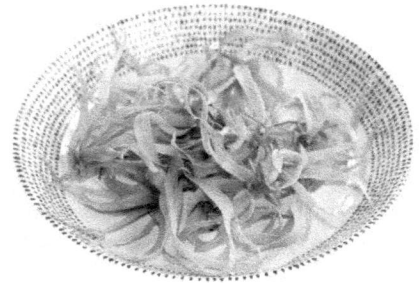

Mix 3 drops of valerian essential oil with 5 drops of ylang-ylang. Put it to you're the water that you will be using when you are going to take a bath.

Lavender and Peppermint Essential Oil Blend Recipe

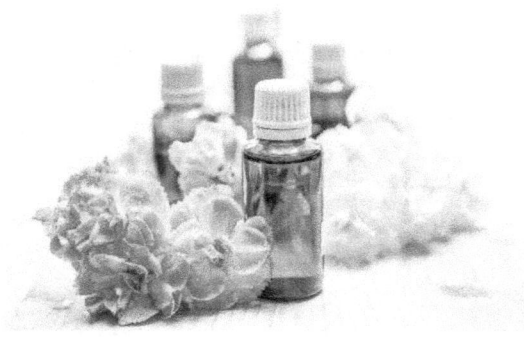

Mix 5 drops of lavender with 3 drops of peppermint essential oil or place it in a diffuser or water that you use when taking a bath.

Lavender and Chamomile Essential Oil Blend Recipe

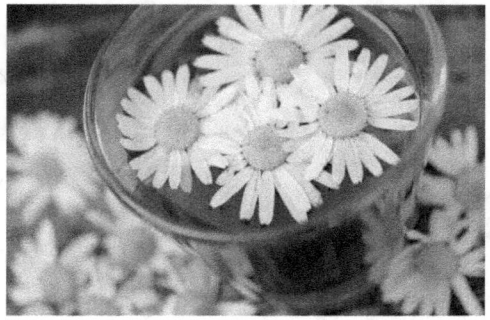

This recipe is good for any kinds of stress just mix 5 drops of lavender essential oil with 4 drops of chamomile oil. Just inhale it whenever you want to or put it on the water that you use in taking a bath.

Essential Oil Blend Recipes for Anxiety

Mix the succeeding essential oils:

Chamomile (16 drops)

Bergamot (2 drops)

Lavender (7 drops)

Geranium (7 drops)

Citrus (8 drops)

How to do it?

Place 2 tbsp of course sea salt in a container.

Place the blends inside it.

Blend them completely and cover it afterward.

Inhale this recipe three times up to 6 times a day to help you resolve your migraine problems.

Chapter 2 – Essential Oil Recipes for Relaxation

There are times when we feel that we are exhausted from the everyday work that we do because of that our energies are drained throughout our body. This is the primary reasons why we look for ways on how to rejuvenate ourselves to bring back the energy loss from the tasks that we do. One way is through the use of essential oils because it is all natural and very effective on its purpose.

Throughout the years a lot of essential oil blend recipes are created to help us relax and soothe our minds for us to function much better whenever needed. Here are some of the recipes that you can make at the comforts of your own home.

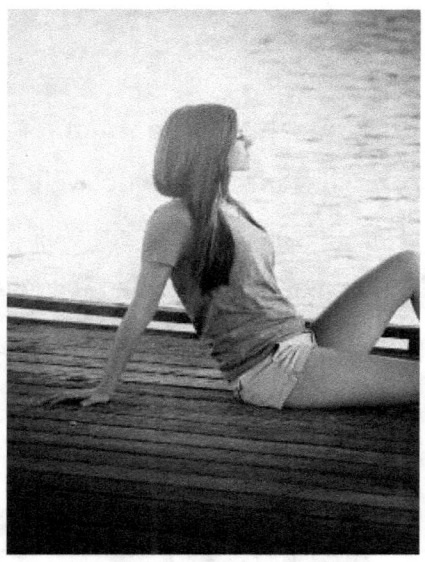

Lavender and Chamomile Blend

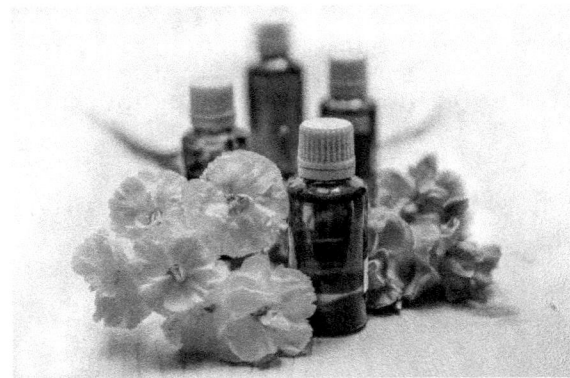

Lavender is popular among the most mainstream and flexible essential oils because it has fragrant healing benefits that can improve your general wellbeing. Since it is it can be used to beautify our skin, heal certain diseases, and restore our health.

What's more? it is also good for the development and maintenance of our brain. Lavender effects the mind similar to what medicines do. When you blend it with chamomile - another essential oil that quiets the nerves - the unwinding boosting properties are much tougher. Chamomile has been demonstrated to battle nervousness and wretchedness.

Lavender and Bergamot

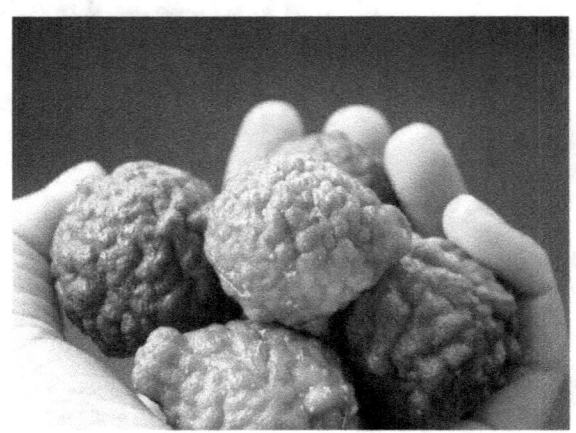

In the event that you are attempting to loosen up because of an unpleasant day, you need fragrant healing that will bring you back on track. In the event that you already have some lavender, add bergamot to add more zen to the recipe. Studies show different fragrance based treatment benefits; bergamot catches the enormous three for advancing mental unwinding, lessening your circulatory strain, pulse, and feeling of anxiety. It likewise mitigates physical agony that can meddle with genuine feelings of serenity.

Lavender, Bergamot, Frankincense, and Cedarwood

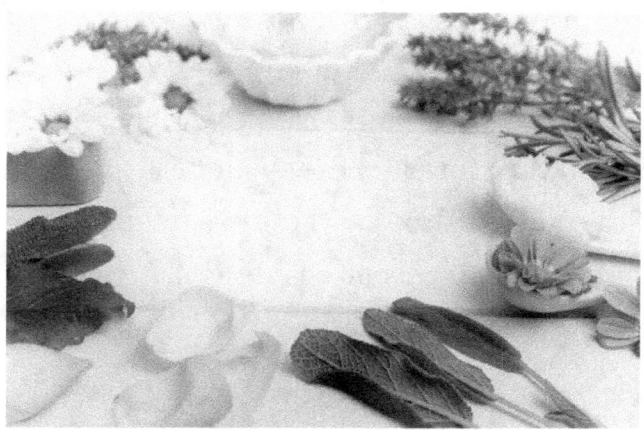

Its been logically demonstrated that, with fragrance-based treatment, you don't need to compromise your magnificence rest. As indicated by different medical professionals, an amazing tranquilizer includes blending bergamot, lavender, frankincense, and cedarwood in a jug. You can even test these oils independently to check whether they help balance your sleep deprivation.

Lemon and Eucalyptus

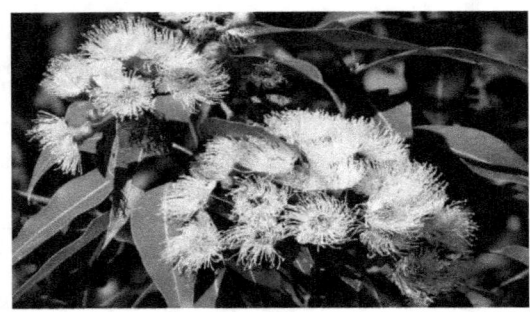

The failure to unwind can prompt interminable pressure and unstable overall health. Fortunately, the blend of lemon and eucalyptus can help mitigate your cold and sinus disease. Lemon is a phenomenal decongestant with antiviral properties, while eucalyptus encourages breathing through a stuffy nose.

Steaming your face with a towel set over your head and bowl of boiling water is unwinding in itself. Include a couple of drops of these oils for a quieting knowledge that will soothe a lot of your dilemmas regarding your health.

Frankincense, Cedarwood, and Chamomile

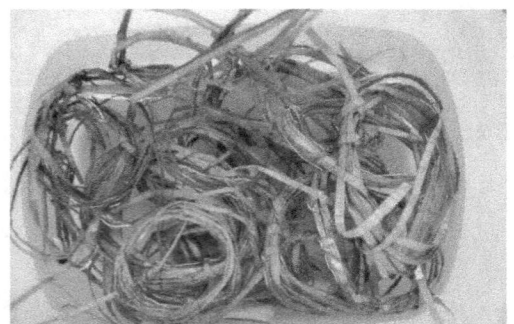

When you can't release it, attempt frankincense. This essential oil has been utilized for a considerable length of time to help individuals ponder. At the point when matched with cedarwood and chamomile, it is significantly increasingly strong in calming the brain.

Chapter 3 – Essential Oil Recipes For Healing

Believe it or not, the best essential oils that we know today are the latest in plant-based treatments. To be reasonable, ancient people practiced various distillation strategies, however, the essential oils that were removed hundreds of years prior were really different from are accessible to us today.Nevertheless, they all contained essential oils and extremely successful at avoiding and any unforeseen sickness.

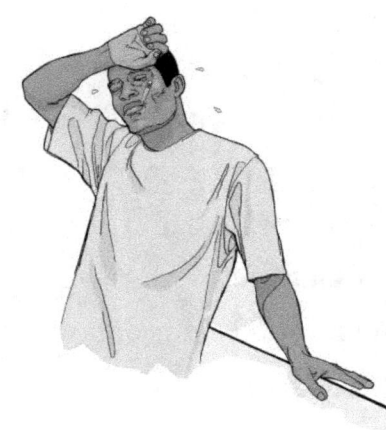

It is said that ancient people were delighted in by those in old Cyprus, Egypt and Pompeii who originally utilized herbs with refining strategies going back 3,500 B.C. This insight cruised over the Mediterranean and clearly achieved Hippocrates, who used fragrance based treatment to their immune systems a couple of hundreds of years before the happening to Christ.

As technology exchanged force to be reckoned with, the method of utilizing the best essential oils for healing from Greece went to Rome, who preferred fragrant healing and aromas.

Master the art of blending essential oils at the comforts of your own home! To help you achieve your wellbeing objectives with fundamental oils if it's not too much trouble make certain to set aside the effort to gain proficiency with the basics of aroma based treatment. The best essential oils for healing are composed of various particles that each convey various impacts on the body.

Here is the rundown of the best essential oils to use for healing

Clove (Eugenia Caryophyllata)

Clove essential oil is generally utilized as a disinfectant for infections mostly the oral ones and to wipe out a wide range of organisms to keep ailment under control. It is known to combat a lot of bacteria such as E. coli and furthermore applied significant power over Staph aureus and Pseudomonas aeruginosa which are two microscopic organisms that are the main causes of pneumonia and skin contaminations.

Eucalyptus Globulus

This essential oil is used mostly by the Aborigines for most ailments in their tribe, eucalyptus is an effective antibacterial, antispasmodic, and antiviral oil. Like clove basic oil, eucalyptus basic oil has a significant effect over Staph contaminations. Did you know that when Staph aureus comes into contact with eucalyptus oil, the dangerous bacteria have totally lost control within a span of 15 minutes!

Frankincense

This essential oil has been utilized with much success in treating issues identified with bodily functions, immune system, oral wellbeing, respiratory concerns, and stress.

Lavender

Know for its alleviating and calming properties, lavender is great for quickening the recuperating time for wounds, stings, and various type of injuries. It is loaded with cancer prevention properties. It is also assessed for its capacity to treat diabetes and anxiety in rodents.

Lemon

Different citrus fundamental oils are broadly used to have healthy nodes, to revive slow, dull skin and as a bug repellent.

Chapter 4 – Essential Oil Recipes for Sleep

Diffusing essential oils for a good rest is one of the main things that got me interested in the world of essential oils.

Like most of us, I used to wake up 1 to 2 times each night. I'd hear the pooch strolling around, or my partner would turn over, or my psyche would race with every one of the things I needed to do the following day. I just couldn't appear to get the rest I desire. I was constantly worn out the next day because I did not get the sleeping hours that I need.

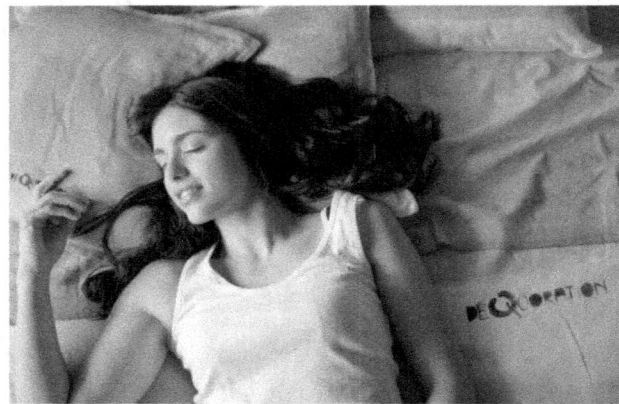

So this is when I try to experiment in using essential oils. I put 4 to 6 drops of lavender basic oil in a diffuser on the surface of my bed. Turned the diffuser on. Lie into my bed and floated off to rest.

Next thing I realized that it relieved the symptoms that I am experiencing before. I had rested straight during that time for an entire 9 hours "In any case, how could this be?" I thought it was just a coincidence.

So I attempted it again the following night. I topped off my diffuser with faucet water, and once more, I put a couple of drops of lavender essential oil in my diffuser. I transformed it on and went straight into my bed. Once more, I slept soundly as the night progressed, not awakening until I regained my consciousness back at 6:00.

There are many fundamental oils that help the psyche and body unwind My preferred essential oils that help an incredible night's rest are lavender, cedarwood, vetiver, marjoram, frankincense, bergamot, sandalwood, Roman chamomile, patchouli, and orange.

Lavender

It is generally utilized for its calming properties. It facilitates pressure and initiates unwinding.

Cedarwood

The warm and woody fragrance that is both establishing and quieting, advancing an incredible night's rest

Vetiver

This grass has a rich, fascinating smell that is really great for manipulating your moods.

Marjoram

It has a warm fragrance that quiets and lets you diminish pressure and other types of anxiousness.

Roman Chamomile

It has a sweet botanical fragrance is quieting and alleviating to the brain and body, making it a standout amongst the frequently utilized essential oils for rest

Wild Orange

It's sweet citrus fragrance and, similar to bergamot, wild orange is an adaptogen that can be empowering or calming, contingent upon what your body needs

Patchouli

The musky aroma is establishing and great for managing your feelings

Hawaiian Sandalwood

It has a rich, sweet and woody fragrance imparts quiet and unwinding. It's alleviating fragrance decreases pressure, advances enthusiastic prosperity, and has a thoughtful impact.

Recipe # 1

Lavender essential oil (2 drops)

Cedarwood essential oil (2 drops)

Recipe #2

Bergamot essential oil (4 drops)

Lavender essential oil (5 drops)

Recipe #3

Lavender essential oil (2 drops)

Wild orange essential oil (2 drops)

Recipe #4

Lavender essential oil (3 drops)

Vetiver essential oil (3 drops)

Marjoram essential oil (3 drops)

Recipe #5

Roman chamomile essential oil (4 drops)

Bergamot essential oil (3 drops)

Frankincense essential oil (3 drops)

Recipe #6

Grounding blend essential oil (4 drops)

Lavender essential oil (3 drops)

Roman chamomile essential oil (3 drops)

Recipe #7

Lavender essential oil (3 drops)

Roman chamomile essential oil (3 drops)

Marjoram essential oil (3 drops)

Recipe #8

Patchouli essential oil (3 drops)

Wild orange essential oil (2 drops)

Frankincense essential oil (3 drops)

Recipe #9

Vetiver essential oil (4 drops)

Lavender essential oil (4 drops)

Frankincense essential oil (3 drops)

Recipe #10

Lavender essential oil (4 drops)

Vetiver essential oil (4 drops)

Recipe #11

Vetiver essential oil (4 drops)

Calming blend essential oil (4 drops)

Recipe #12

3 drops patchouli essential oil

3 drops sandalwood essential oil

Chapter 5 – Essential Oil Recipes for Hair Growth

Another advantage of essential oils have is its capacity to enhance our hair. Various oils can do everything from helping the hair to sparkle and to become stronger.

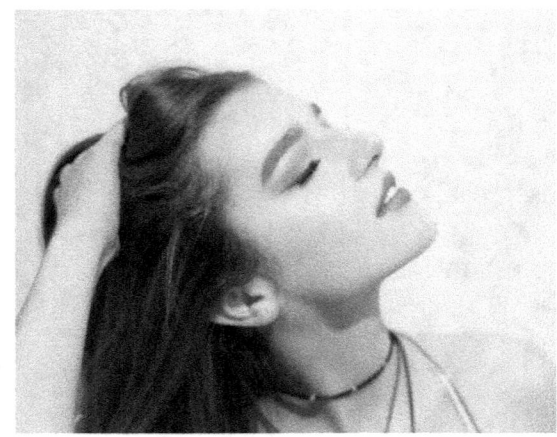

Here are the most effective essential oils for your hair:

Lavender

It can accelerate hair development. Realizing that lavender oil has properties that can create the development of cells and lessen pressure, scientists on one creature examine found that this oil had the option to produce quicker hair development in mice.

It also has antimicrobial and antibacterial properties, which can improve scalp wellbeing. Blend a few drops of lavender oil into 3 tablespoons of bearer oil, similar to olive oil or softened coconut oil, and apply it generously to your scalp. Let it sit for 10 minutes before washing it out and shampooing as you typically would. You can do this a few times each week.

Peppermint

Peppermint oil can cause a cool, shivering inclination while having a good circulation on the portion of your body that you will apply it. This can help promote the growth of new hair.

One research found that peppermint oil, when utilized on mice, expanded the number of follicles for more opportunity of growing hair. Blend 3 drops of peppermint basic oil with your preferred carrier oil. Backrub into your scalp, and let it sit for 5 minutes before washing out altogether with cleanser and conditioner.

Rosemary

If you need to improve both hair thickness and hair development, rosemary oil is a great choice because of its capacity to enhance our cells.

Blend a few drops of rosemary oil with olive or coconut oil, and apply it to your scalp. Let it sit for 10 minutes before washing it out with cleanser. Do this two times in seven days for more a desirable outcome.

Cedarwood

This essential oil is thought to promote hair development and diminish the usual male pattern baldness by adjusting the oil-producing organs in the scalp. It also has antifungal and antibacterial properties, which can treat various conditions that may add to dandruff or balding.

If you will put it into a blend with lavender, rosemary, and cedarwood it was found to diminish male pattern baldness in those with alopecia areata. Blend a couple of drops of cedarwood essential oil with 1 tbsp of carrier oil of your preference. Backrub into your scalp, and abandon it on for 10 minutes before washing it out.

Lemongrass basic oil

Dandruff can be a big problem, and having a dandruff-free scalp is a significant piece of hair wellbeing. Lemongrass oil is a very effective dandruff treatment and it is better if you will add it to your daily regimen. Blend a couple of drops into your shampoo and ensure it's rubbed really well into your scalp.

Chapter 6 – Essential Oil for Cancer and Other Diseases

I stand that one of the most useful types of herbal medicines in the world is essential oils. From triggering tranquility to calming our skin, aids healing and the combat certain illnesses, essential oils gives boundless opportunities to your well-being. I'll just clarify that the utilization of these oils is not just a trend. Essential oils have been used already by our ancestors from the different portions of the world in ancient times.

Nowadays, my family and I utilized these oils in various uses in our everyday life. The purpose of these healing objects is pretty tremendous. I'll put a rundown of it, but some ways we usually utilize essential oils comprise as medicines, for hygiene, detoxification, and etc.Why do we consider all of us must imitate us in utilizing essential oils as a basic necessity.

It's basic. We chose to utilize nonhazardous natural ways that have proven credibility in terms of their advantages, over a complete reliance on the prescribed medicines that are known for their side-effects.

Similarly, we opt to utilize own hygienic items and cleansers that are a great option because you are getting the cleansing power without the harmful chemicals. We get similar or even better outcomes while diminishing the hazards in our very own health.

I often questioned about the essential oils we prefer using to improve our overall health and prevent the formation of cancers, and also how we utilize them. This is the primary reason why I will share it to you so that you can also improve your health just like me and my family with the use of these essential oils.

Frankincense

Frankincense likely could be my absolute favorite essential oil because it fights certain tumors. It is mitigating, for one, which is imperative in the journey to recuperate from a lot of illnesses not only cancer. In particular, frankincense has been appeared to be an intense inhibitor of 5-lipoxygenase, a catalyst in charge of the immune system in the body.

It also helps support resistant capacity and anticipates sickness by duplicating white platelets and balancing invulnerable responses. It additionally improves flow, and decrease the pressure in our body. Oil of frankincense has appeared to contract and tone tissues, which speeds recovery.

Frankincense also appeared to give neurological help, including the capacity to get rid of poisons that may prompt neurological harm.

Nonetheless, it has a few advantages with regards to malignant tumor treatments, including relieving joint inflammation, equalizing hormones, empowering skin wellbeing, and helping assimilation.

Lavender

It has the phytochemicals perillyl liquor and linalool that are proven to drive malignant tumors away from our body.

It minimizes stress and supports the capacity of the immune system to perform better. Sleeping patterns are also improved with the use of this oil. Sadness and nervousness are completely taken away from our senses too. These go towards supporting the immune system in the battling of different illnesses.

Medical research has concluded that lavender essential oil is great in fighting different kinds of bacteria making the people who are using it really healthy.

Myrrh

Myrrh is considered as a very useful essential oil in the world of herbal medicines because it has a lot of incredible healing properties that. As far as disease healing is concerned, myrrh essential oil shows outstanding results in fighting malignant tumors.

It is also known to provide equilibrium in the hormones inside our body, which can be very crucial in healing. Like lavender and frankincense, It is also been utilized as a stress reliever.

Peppermint

It is a miracle oil with a wide scope of advantages. This essential oil's advantages in fighting cancers originate from its phytochemicals limonene, phytochemicals beta-caryophyllene, and beta-pinene, which are known for their effective detoxification properties.

Research says that this essential oil has the capacity to provide cell reinforcement and cancer-fighting agent properties which mostly concentrates on the prevention of tumor growth. It also contains antiangiogenic properties, which keep tumors from building up their own blood supply.

It also has antibacterial properties that make it really advantageous for fighting respiratory infection.

Turmeric

This essential oil has shown that if it is in a concentrated form, is known to battle malignant cells while advancing apoptosis resulting in a cancer-free body.

This very efficient essential oil has different advantages also that includes controlling glucose, help wounds heal rapidly, avert Alzheimer's illness, support you in getting a fit body, and simplicity joint pain.

<u>How to Use Essential Oils for Healing?</u>

Essential oils are so indispensable to my family's life, it's difficult to list each way we are using them! Whatever it may be, here are some top tips for utilizing essential oils in your everyday life.

- Put a drop behind your ears

  On a daily basis, I put myrrh and frankincense behind my ears and on the lymph hubs as a prophylactic (precaution insurance). Lavender or peppermint would be useful for respiratory issues, or basically to unwind. You can rub on the back of the skull, the bosoms, or the bottoms of your feet.

- Use a cool diffuser

  We want to diffuse essential oils all through our home. We do it for included mental lucidity. My office is constantly loaded up with the restorative smells of an assortment of essential oils.

- Massage into the skin

  Some basic oils, similar to peppermint and clove, are exceptionally solid and it will become perfect if you will combine it with other types of oil

- You can utilize a decent quality, natural (ideally cool squeezed) oil like coconut, olive, or jojoba to blend in a couple of drops of your preferred fundamental oil.

  You would then be able to knead this straightforward "body margarine" onto your skin. For somewhat fancier body margarine, utilize a blender to whip strong coconut oil with fundamental oil. Utilize this blend to apply straightforwardly to influenced zones, (for example, with agony, joint pain, or stomach related problems), and for a snappy mind and other medical advantages.

- Ingest Internally

  One of my top pick, because I usually combine essential oils with my soothing beverages what I usually make is a so-called "Peppermint Lemonade."

I basically take 5-10 drops of peppermint essential oil, around twelve drops of lemon (or orange or tangerine oils, contingent upon my temperament), include water, some natural green stevia, and ice in an expansive pitcher. It's a super-quick, solid refreshment that I cherish. It's likewise delectable as a hot drink (utilize hot water and exclude the ice). In case you're simply making one glass at any given moment, utilize just 1 drop of peppermint + 1 drop of citrus oil. You can likewise utilize a couple of drops of essential oils in an unfilled gel container and swallow it.

- Toothpaste

You can make an assortment of individual items utilizing natural essential oils and other non-poisonous substances such as creams, face washes, mouthwash, cleansers. A toothpaste is anything but difficult to make but it proved me wrong because with the use of natural frankincense, myrrh, and coconut oil it became as easy as 1, 2, and 3.

Conclusion

That was a long ride, I hope that you have learned a lot from the essential oil recipes that we have tackled a while ago. Just one piece of advice before we part ways, I suggest that you must be creative when it comes to blending the various essential oils. The primary reason for this is that the recipes of essential oil blends are not just limited to the ones that are listed here because you can actually make one of your own depends on your needs.

Just make sure to study the different oils that are in this book so that the next time you plan to make your own recipe you will know the use of each essential oil which will help you make a very astounding recipe in the future. But before anything else I would like to discuss to you the key points that you should remember if you want to use essential oils.

Quality

This is important to the point that it bears rehashing. Continuously utilize a top-quality, therapeutic essential oil. It ought to be ensured natural, and 100% unadulterated. Check the notoriety of your provider, and guarantee there are no fillers or added substances.

Keep oils from delicate territories

Essential oils are nature's powerhouses. Remember they are 40-50 times stronger than the plant itself. A few oils are progressively "fiery" than others. Some taste superior to other people.

Oregano is one that can consume a bit when you ingest it legitimately. Peppermint requires alert, and generally does best with a transporter oil when applying to the skin. Never apply essential oils to touchy territories of the body, including the private areas or close to your eyes.

You ought to likewise test new oils to guarantee there are no responses before applying too generously.

You can begin by completing a sniff trial of the oil in the jug. In an instance that appears to be fine, at that point apply a spot of oil to within your wrist or arm, include a drop of oil and hold on to check whether there is any redness, tingling, or swelling. Everyone's body is unique so you may need to attempt various oils to see which ones feel best to you.

Do not heat up oils

You've most likely observed or even have one of those oil burners for utilizing essential oils. What you can be sure of is that warming these oils decimates their healing properties. It's in every case best to utilize a cool diffuser. These are abundant and monetarily evaluated on the web.

Keep out of Children

Continuously be mindful when utilizing essential oils with kids. Dispersion is the most secure. For direct application, it's critical to weakening the more grounded oils, particularly with a decent oil. When making body spreads or back rub oils for kids, utilize 1 drop of essential oil to 4 tablespoons of other oils.

This will weaken the essential oil enough to make it progressively in the middle of the road and more secure for your kid. Be mindful so as not to put close to the eyes and dependably complete an allergy test first.

One word is very important in creating your own essential oil recipe which is "creativity" always apply that when you plan to make a recipe. So that's it I wish you good luck to your future endeavors.

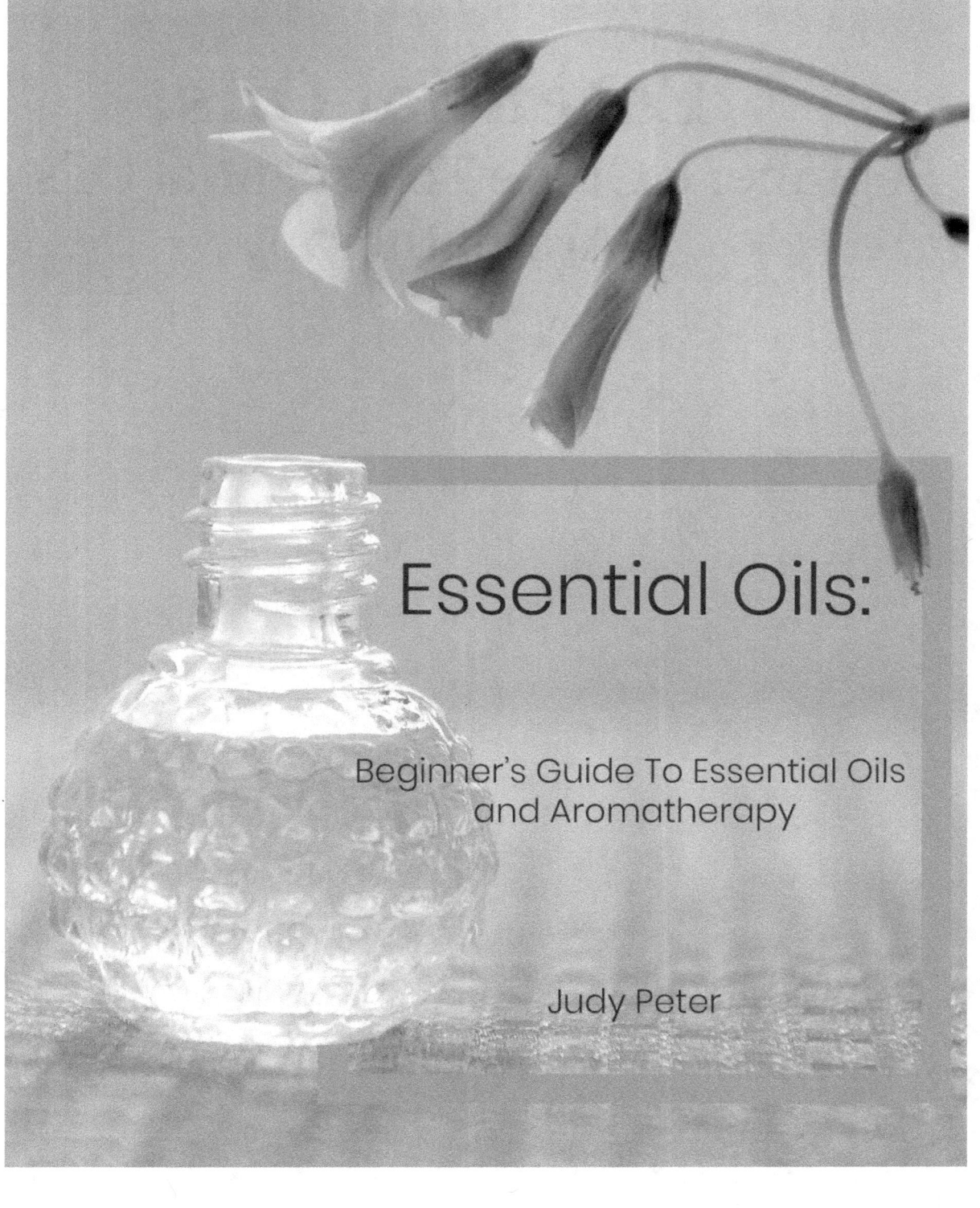

Essential Oils:

Beginner's Guide To Essential Oils and Aromatherapy

Judy Peter

Essential Oils:
Beginner's Guide To Essential Oils and Aromatherapy

Introduction: The Soothing Satisfaction of Essential Oil

Essential oils are essentially just a much more concentrated batch of plant oils already found in nature. Lemon essential oil for example, is simply the natural oil extracted from a lemon in a much more powerfully condensed form. This oil is usually created by way of distillation—produced through hot steam. This method makes sure that the most potent batch of oil is created with the least amount of effort.

The main essence of the oils once extracted are usually paired with a base or "carrier" oil and then further refined for human consumption. If your oil is not mixed with a carrier agent, caution must be exercised as some essential oils have been known to be so powerful that they cause irritation to exposed skin.

It is for this reason that diluting just a few drops in a carrier oil are usually recommended. People have come to greatly benefit from the use of specific essential oils whether by simply inhaling them through aromatherapy or rubbing them directly into the skin during a massage.

Aromatherapy in particular has shown much promise when it comes to improving mood and other mental conditions. Our nose as it turns out is very much connected to our emotions—the nose actually links right up to glands in our limbic system such as the hippocampus which is a major center for both our emotions and our all too often limited—attention spans. By simply inhaling certain chemical compounds our moods can be lifted and concentration can be improved.

The practice of aromatherapy through the use of essential oils has been used for thousands of years. It is for this reason that many ancient religions use incense during their religious services because the sweet aroma of the incense is often viewed as necessary for bringing the congregants into just the right mental state. Those who participated in these time-honored rituals knew just how fulfilling they were. But you don't have to wait until the next mass to benefit from aromatherapy.

This book provides you with detailed recipes of essential oils that you can put together in your own home. So, get ready. Because now you too are about to discover the soothing satisfaction that these essential oils can offer.

Chapter 1: How Aromatherapy Works

The nose of course is the organ that fosters our sense of smell but it runs much deeper than that. The nose is actually a bit of a messenger for the other important systems of our body, playing a major role in our daily function. So, having that said, before we delve into our aromatherapy recipes, let's take a brief look on just how it is that the nose works.

Basic Function of the Nose

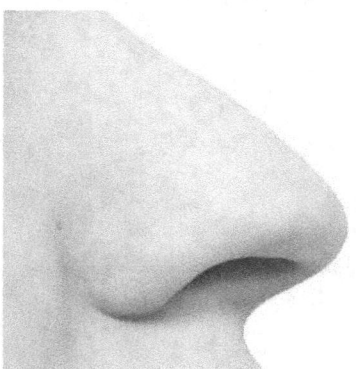

The nose is part of a complicated sensory system in our body which stand on the front line to sort out all of the chemical compounds that we are bombarded with on a daily basis. Whether those compounds are molecules rising up from a freshly cooked steak, or the smell of your car's smoking radiator.

Our nose alerts us ahead of time to what we are about to get into. The nose is important as an information system, informing us of what we are up against. But it does more than alert us to smelly things nearby, it also processes those same chemical compounds that we inhale, taking specific smell molecules and combining them to receptors that influence our mood, memory, and emotion. You see, our nose plays a much bigger role than most of us care to realize.

Despite alerting us to strong odors and fragrances, the nose is constantly working on even the most subconscious of levels influencing our mood and temperament. Just about everywhere we go we encounter miniscule little smell molecules are wafting up our nostrils. After passing into our nostrils, they dock with special chemical sensory receptors and impart some very specific information to your body as well as providing the receptors with a very specific stimulus.

That stimulus could be for energy, to go to sleep, or even to raise the metabolism —all depending on what the chemical compound has to impart upon these nasal receptors. And just think about it, all of these complex exchanges occur faster than you can smell the afternoon popcorn! This is just the basic function of our nose at work.

Application Methods

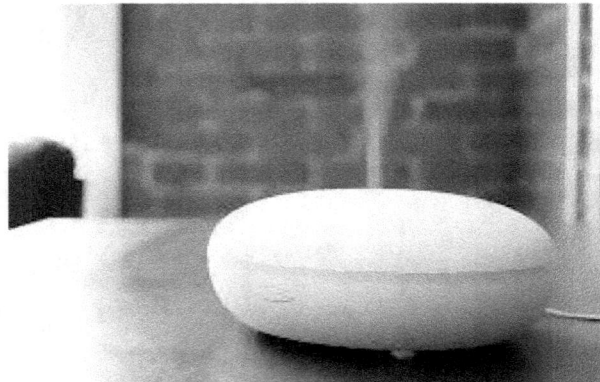

Now that we know how the nose works, let's look at some application methods for aromatherapy. The most basic way to use essential oils for aromatherapy would be just to inhale their scent right out of the bottle. I personally have done this myself to treat my asthma with a variety of essential oils I keep around, such as peppermint and frankincense.

In those moments that I feel tightness in my chest and receive the distinct indication of a bad episode of asthma coming on, I just pull out one of the bottles take the lid off and breathe in as deep as I possibly can

For a quick fix, this method of application is helpful. And without any extra equipment or elaborate preparation, benefits can be gleaned. But although useful, this method leaves much to be desired. For a more powerful effect, you could simply deposit a few drops of the oil in a container of boiling or near boiling water. This water can be heated up either through the use of a tea kettle or simply by placing a container filled with water into the microwave and heating it up for a few minutes on high.

However, it is that you do it, as soon as the oil hits the hot water it will rise up as steam. Once the steam starts to flow, simply lean over the container and breathe in the aroma. The most effective way of using these oils in aromatherapy however would be to actually purchase and use a diffuser. The diffuser is an appliance that mechanically spreads the aroma of essential oils through the air through steam. This is the basic gist of how aromatherapy works.

Chapter 2: Aromatic Anxiety Relief Recipes

Anxiety is a big problem in the modern world. We are all busy and rushing from one place to the next. Not only that, even in our free time most of us tend to be constantly looking at a screen—whether its our laptop, tablet or phone, we are constantly fiddling with a technological device in order to keep up. But all of this constant stimulation is causing our brains to go into hyperdrive.

So much so in fact, that the next time you are forced to look away from your phone and do absolutely nothing, the adjustment can be downright painful. Simply having to stare up at a red traffic light for example, and you find yourself becoming increasingly anxious for that said light to turn green. The mind that is used to constantly running is now forced to sit still with nothing to do, and it doesn't like it!

Having trouble putting your overworked mind into standby mode for mundane tasks is an indication that things are getting out of whack. It is a clear sign of an overloaded system in need of some pure and simple anxiety relief! The recipes presented in this chapter are geared to help you breathe out that stress, worry and anxiety and breathe in the aroma of calm and soothing essential oils.

Rose Essential Oil

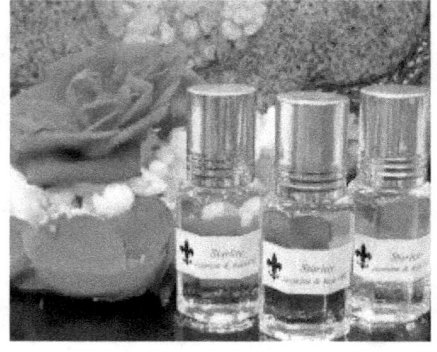

Rose essential oil comes directly from fresh cut roses. If anyone has ever asked you to slow down to "stop and smell the roses", it's because the scent of this flower is able to put people at ease simply by smelling it.

It is for this reason that essential rose oil, which is basically just a much more highly concentrated batch of that same aroma from a fresh cut rose, is so effective at lessoning the symptoms that result from of an anxious and overworked mind. Rose essential oil is so powerful in fact, that routine regimens of it has been shown to actually calm the heart and reduce the incidence of high blood pressure in the body.

If you need a natural way to calm your racing heart and mind, this oil could be just what you are looking for. It opens airways, slows the pulse and alleviates any lingering brain fog from the mind. In order to create your own batch of essential rose oil for aromatherapy, just add a few drops of rose oil to your choice of carrier oil and burn it as incense or run it through a good diffuser.

Allow yourself to then gradually inhale the aroma for a few hours and you will be feeling great. Yes, it truly is a good thing when we to take some time to smell the roses! Try this blend of rose essential oil today!

Geranium Essential Oil

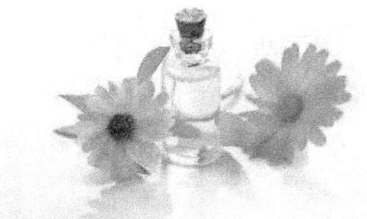

The Geranium flower is great when it comes to relieving anxiety. Geranium oil is actually very similar to rose oil in composition but for those that are interested—geranium oil is usually a whole heck of a lot cheaper than rose oil. So, having that said, for a cheaper yet still highly effective anxiety reliever this essential oil could be your go-to source.

Geranium oil is indeed an essential ingredient. This oil produces a very nice scent that fills the room with a gentle almost citrus-like aroma. Just place 4 or 5 drops into a good carrier oil, and toss it into an incense burner or proper diffuser, and you are good to go. Give yourself 30 to 40 minutes to breathe in the aroma that is produced. For an extra boost you could also add 2 drops of clary sage oil. Just breathe in the aroma until you feel yourself begin relax!

Bergamot and Lavender Essential Oil Mix

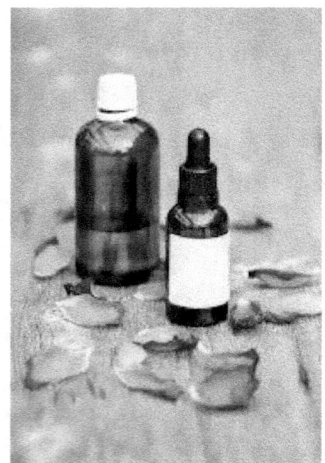

The reason why both Bergamot and Lavender are crucial ingredients when it comes to relieving anxiety is due to a little something called "linalyl acetate". This chemical has been shown to relax both the body and the mind as soon as our nose encounters it.

This combination of bergamot and lavender also provides us with a rather distinctive and pleasing aroma as well. Just add a couple drops of Bergamot along with at least one drop of lavender into a proper carrier oil, distribute to an incense burner, and allow the sweet scent to fill the room. The feeling is almost immediate, and you will be feeling better in no time. Go ahead and give it try!

Neroli Essential Oil

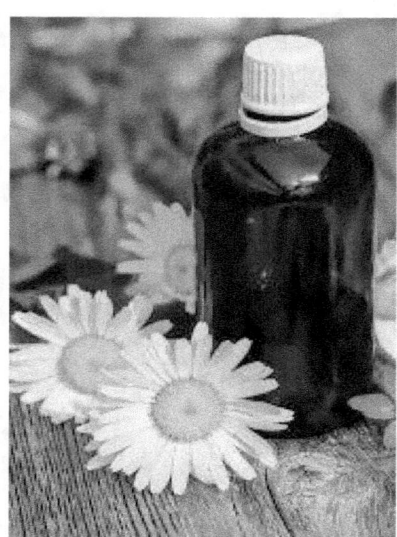

Neroli essential oil is a true workhouse when it comes to essential oils. This powerful and refreshing essential oil has been known to actually slow down the quickened pulse, and bring clarity to the troubled mind.

This calming and classy oil refreshes the entire system simply from breathing in its aroma. Neroli originates from the Seville orange tree. It is actually the orange peels from which neroli oil is extracted. The name is said to have its origins in the Italian town of Nerola where this essential oil was widely manufactured and used by the locals.

This essential oil was used in religious ceremonies as incense as well as by those simply wishing to take the edge off of their own edginess. And don't just take my word for it—take the word of science. Because this oil has been shown in several scientific studies to the improve moods of those who partake of it.

One of the most recent in fact had a group of women dealing with depression and anxiety breathe in neroli as a form of aromatherapy while another group of women breathed in just basic almond oil. Without being told which type of oil they were breathing, time and time again, the group of women who inhaled neroli saw a relief of their symptoms. Whereas the women who partook of just basic almond oil so no difference.

This study clearly indicates a connection between neroli and the alleviation of anxiety. In order to start your own aromatherapy regimen with neroli, simply add 4 or 5 drops to a carrier oil and inhale as incense, or place a few drops with a cup of water into your diffuser. You will feel a lot better for it!

Frankincense Essential Oil

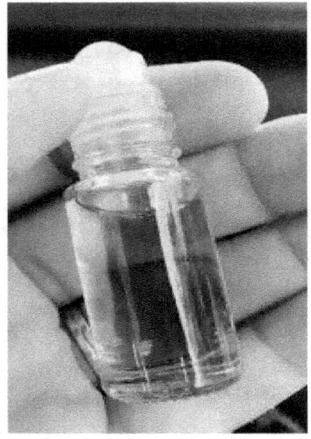

Hailing from the African continent, this ancient essential oil has been held as a prized possession the world over, for literally thousands of years. And for good reason. The rare chemicals within this essential oil have the ability to relieve stress and bring back mental clarity like no other.Just about anyone feeling down in the dumps will feel remarkably better once the fragrance of frankincense has been introduced.

It is for this reason that religions all over the globe have burned incense of frankincense during religious ceremonies. And if you can recall your Christmas nativity, frankincense and myrrh played quite a pivotal role there as well. Frankincense in some places was actually valued to be worth more than gold. Demonstrating that the ancients placed just as much worth on having proper mental clarity as we do today.

Because the aroma of this oil has quite a way of easing away stress and bringing the mind to a proper state of balance. So. without further ado, let's get started on your own batch of frankincense. Just add a few drops to a good base, carrier oil, place inside your incense burner or diffuser and allow the aroma to gradually release in a centralized part of your home. Now get ready to breathe in the majestic relaxation that only this powerful and potent essential oil can bring about.

Cypress Essential Oil

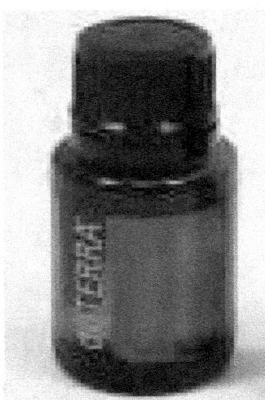

Coming from the cypress tree—this essential oil has long been prized for its ability to reduce the stress in those that come to use it. The oil itself is extracted through a process of steam distillation aimed at the tree's branches and needles.

The oil has a powerful sedative like quality that creates a great feeling of relaxation without making you drowsy. But the aroma of this oil not only calms you down it also puts you at ease with a truly content feeling. The best way to use cypress essential oil is to mix 5 drops of it with a cup of hot water and pour it right into your diffuser

You could also simply add the mix to a hot bath if you would prefer. Just give it about an hour or so to work and soon you will be feeling relaxed and at peace. If you are indeed suffering from stress and anxiety the essential oil recipes presented in this chapter are a great resource for you to have on hand.

Chapter 3: Essential Oil Recipes for Energy and Focus

In the non-stop world of today it seems that we are staying up later and setting our alarm clocks back earlier, and yet we are still never quite seeming to find the time or energy needed to stay on task. Our minds aimlessly wander and we find ourselves missing deadlines as we get stuck in the drift.

For most the go-to solution for this problem would be a good cup of coffee but too much coffee can take its physiological toll, leading to sleeplessness, irritability and anxiety. Is there a healthier alternative? Look no farther than the soothing scent of essential oils! Many of us could use a little mental boost when it comes to our energy and focus—here in this chapter we will show you how to do just that!

<u>Lemon Essential Oil</u>

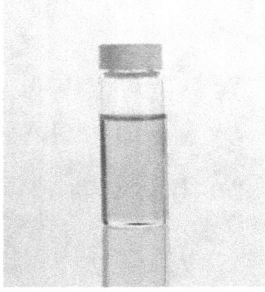

Lemons are one of nature's wonder fruits. Lemons are good for a wide variety of purposes and when condensed down into an essential oil their attributes become even more pronounced. Lemon essential oil as soon as it is inhaled works to relax both breathing and blood vessels, slowing down the heart rate and bringing about a natural sense of calm and contentment.

If you are feeling stressed out and could use a little boost, you really need to give this recipe a try. It's quick, it's painless, and most importantly—it's effective! The ingredients are quite simple, just add anywhere between 5 to 7 drops of lemon essential oil into a good incense burner or diffuser and breath in the resulting steam over the next few hours. It's a weekend getaway without ever leaving the house!

Peppermint and Cinnamon Essential Oil Mix

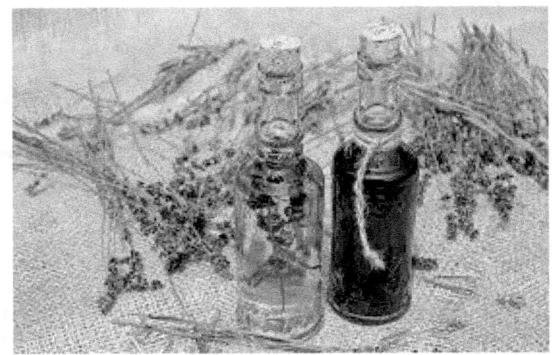

Peppermint is yet another powerful essential oil that serves a wide variety of purposes yet in particular, this oil has been found to be quite a bit of use in the form of an energy booster. If you have ever breathed in the full, natural aroma of peppermint you can probably attest to the fact that it tends to draw in your senses.

Cinnamon complements peppermint and enhances its powerful draw. Keeping that in mind, here is a special blend just for you. In order to create this mix, you will need to add 5 drops of peppermint oil and 4 drops of cinnamon oil to a carrier oil. Once mixed together, you can burn as incense or in your diffuser. Breathe in deep because the effects are almost immediate.

Rosemary Essential Oil

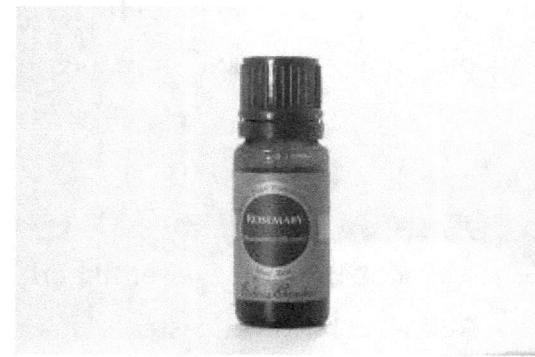

Rosemary is a great stress buster and also helps to improve our concentration and focus. A regular regimen of this essential oil helps us to make the best of our day as our increased attention span gets to work. You will find that incessant worry slipping away as you focus on the most immediate task at hand. And its powerful! Just a few drops of this stuff will do you! Add just 3 or 4 drops of this oil to a carrier base, place into your incense burner or diffuser and you are ready to roll!

The aroma produced has a pleasant, woodsy kind of feel to it. Think of that refreshing feeling when you step onto a forest trail in a nature park and you will have an idea of the pleasing aroma that rosemary essential oil can produce.

Eucalyptus Essential Oil

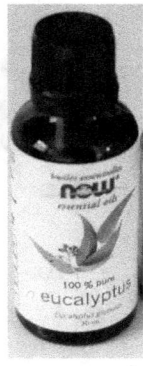

Eucalyptus provides what has been described as a cool and refreshing aroma. The act of breathing in this oil provides us with an energetic boost that resets and reboots our entire system. The chemical compounds released bond directly with special receptors in the nose and get to work.

Inhalation of the fumes produced by this essential oil has also been known to reduce the onset of headaches as well as relieve congested sinuses, making it an excellent choice for allergy sufferers.

As it turns out, Eucalyptus essential oil also doubles as an antibacterial agent and by burning it in a room, the resulting residue works to clear out any pesky bacteria that may be present, including dangerous hard to reach molds. So, as well as keeping you alert and focused, this essential oil also keeps your home and health in pretty good shape as well.

In order to create your own batch of eucalyptus essential oil just add about 6 drops of eucalyptus oil to a ½ a cup of water mixed with 2 tablespoons of cornstarch. Mix these ingredients together well and add to an incense burner or diffuser. Allow the aroma to fill the room you are in and breathe in the aroma. Eucalyptus is quite a refreshing blend that will have you back for more!

Lime Essential Oil

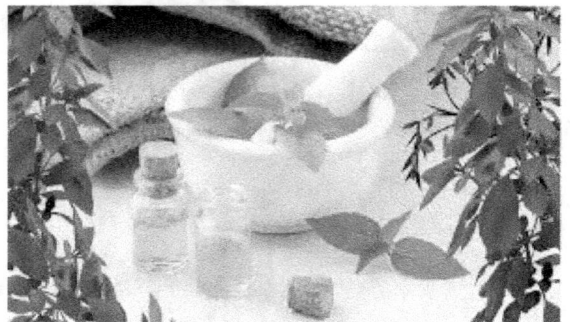

Lime essential oil is good by itself or combined with the aforementioned lemon essential oil. Lime just like lemon is good at uplifting mood and boosting general energy levels of those who use it. It has a very clean scent and can be used just about anywhere. Be warned however that lime does tend to have a rather powerful aroma and having that said not everyone likes the smell of lime.

This is more a demonstration of personal preference than anything else however, and if the aroma is pleasing to you, it does indeed do well to waken up the senses. In order to give yourself your own dose of lime essential oil, simply place a few drops of lime oil along with ½ a cup of water into a diffuser and give yourself at least an hour to slowly breath in the aroma as it diffuses out into the surrounding environment.

Pine Essential Oil

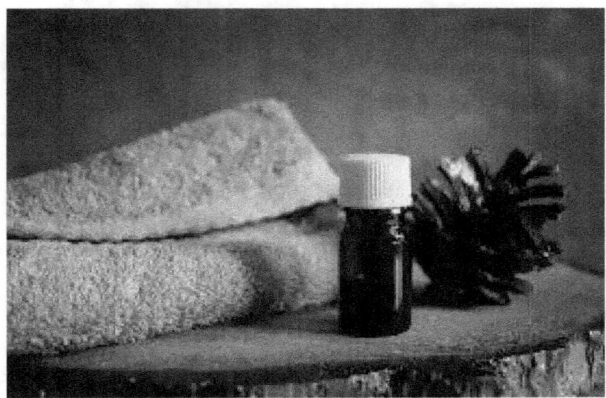

As pure as a pine tree—pine essential oil provides a pristine blend of energy enhancing aroma! This essential oil can be mixed with cedar for extra effect or just used as is. Take 4 or 5 drops and place them in your diffuser along with a good carrier oil and breath in deep! After the first 10 to 15 minutes you should be feeling alert and focused. Try some pine essential oil today!

Chapter 4: Essential Oil Recipes for Immune Health

Our health is everything. If we are not feeling at our best our work as well as our downtime will both suffer for it. And what is it that protects and guarantees our health more than anything else? The biggest vanguard of our well-being will always be our immune system.

You can think of our immune system as an invisible shield that keeps out harmful biological agents. If that wall of immunity begins to be compromised these agents will begin to break through and wreak havoc on our health. Fortunately for us, there are many essential oils that can help to boost our immune health. Keep reading to find out more about them!

<u>Ginger Essential Oil</u>

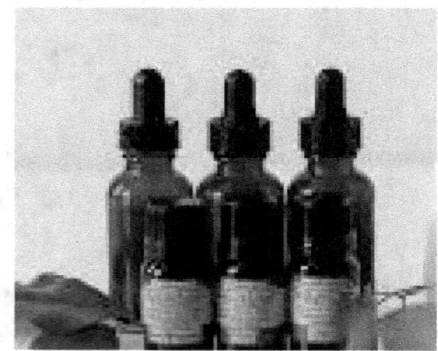

Ginger essential oil is a great immune booster. Ginger is said to have originated in China and since has spread to many other parts of the world. The oil itself is usually extracted from the root of the ginger plant. Ginger has been used for thousands of years as an additive to meals due to both its flavor and its seeming ability of aiding the stomach to digest food.

Ginger oil has many anti-inflammatory properties and these properties work well to boost a faltering immune system. Just add a few drops of ginger essential oil to a carrier oil, add a tablespoon of water and you are good to go. Place this mix into an incense burner or diffuser, sit back and inhale the resulting aroma.

Oregano Essential Oil

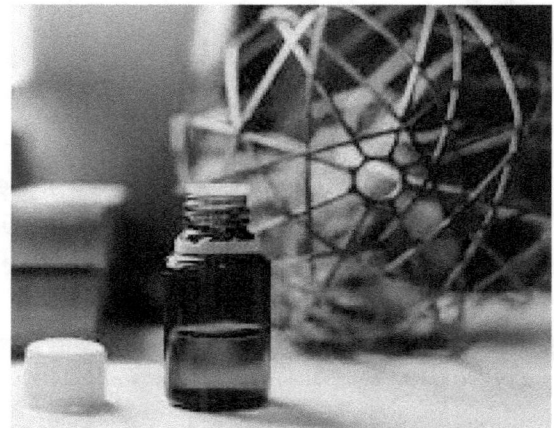

Most of us are probably primarily familiar with oregano as an ingredient in our food, but trust me, it does much more than simply enrich the flavor of our pasta! Oregano contains something called thymol and another little something called carvacrol. Both of these elements are known immune boosters.

Oregano oil comes with plenty of antioxidants that help to ensure that the body keeps a good equilibrium when it comes to keeping out harmful biological agents. Add 5 drops of oregano oil to ½ a cup of water, and mix with a carrier oil. Place inside your incense burner or diffuser. And that's it, folks!

Saffron Essential Oil

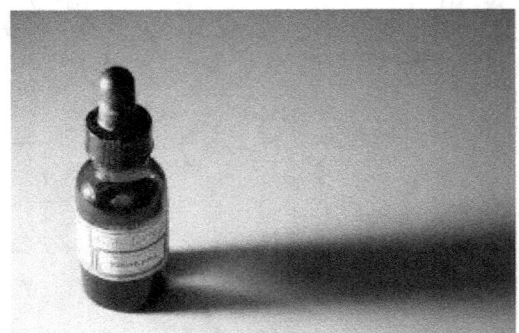

An exotic spice found in the climes of Southern Europe; saffron is one of the most sought-after herbs on the planet. Just one pound of saffron can at times cost over a thousand dollars. Not to worry however folks, because its true—just a dab of this stuff will do you! This oil is so potent that just a few drops should do the trick.

Taken from the stems of the saffron plant; the essential oil produced does wonders for the overtaxed immune system. Saffron can actually help promote a healthier cardiovascular system and boost the metabolic rate of the body which in tur supports a stronger and more robust immune system. Just put two or three drops of Saffron combined with a suitable carrier oil, into your incense burner or diffuser, and you will soon see some pretty nifty results!

Astragalus Essential Oil

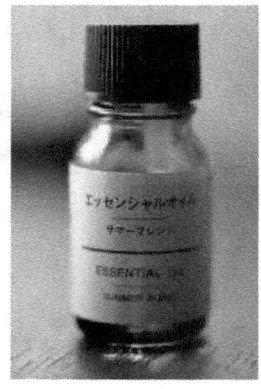

Used for countless centuries by Chinese herbalists, astragalus has been known to strengthen even the weakest of immune systems. The elderly in particular have shown much promising results through regular aromatherapy sessions with astragalus essential oil. So, just where does this immune boosting power come from?

Well—for one thing astragalus has a hefty dose of antioxidants, which are always quite good for stimulating our body's immune system. Astragalus also helps our circulation and cardio function. which in turn helps our body to keep our immune system well regulated and at its best.

So, just add one drop with a cup of water and place them into your diffuser or incense burner. Just a drop or two will do you—let your incense and diffuser do the rest!

Echinacea Essential Oil

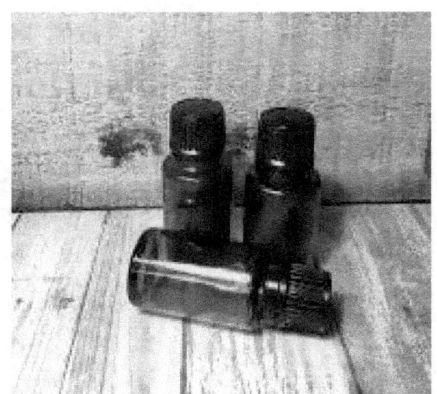

Echinacea has both antiviral and antibiotic properties and as such has been used for thousands of years the world over to aid those that are feeling a bit under the weather.

If you are sick and could use an immune boost, echinacea essential oil would be a good place for you to turn for some relief. The reason for this being that the oil from this plant contain polysaccharides.

What are polysaccharides you might ask? They are special protein building blocks needed by the body, and the reason why they are good for the immune system is due to their ability to activate white blood cells—our bodies mighty gatekeepers and defenders against biological disease.

Having that said, in order to create your own echinacea essential oil treatment, just take 4 drops of echinacea oil, 2 tablespoons of water, and mix with a good carrier oil. Add this to either an incense burner, or a diffuser, give yourself about an hour to breathe in the resulting aroma, and you are ready to go.

Cedar Essential Oil

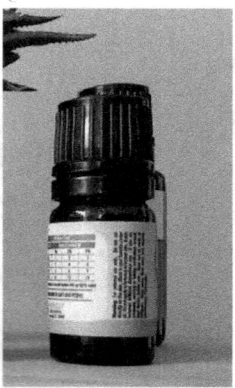

In its raw form, cedar essential oil holds much promise when it comes to boosting the immune system. This oil is obtained through direct steam distillation from pieces of cedar taken directly from a tree.

The trees that they are taken from are typically in cold or mountainous regions. Just think of the Alps and your mind is on the right track of where this oil is naturally found.

The main elements found within cedar are bedta cedrane, alpha cedrane, cedrol, widdrol, and thujopsene—all of which are known immune boosters. Their names may be hard to pronounce, but their effect is nothing short of extraordinary. So, let's get you started. For this recipe take 3 drops of cedar oil and mix it with 1 drop of cypress and 1 drop of rosemary. Add this mixture to diffuser, and allow the aroma to fill the air.

Orange Essential Oil

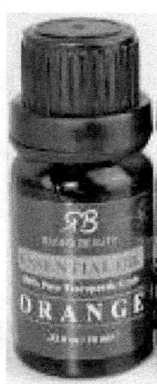

If you have ever had a cold in your life, then someone somewhere has more than likely recommended you to drink some orange juice. And there is most certainly a good reason for that since oranges are a well-known immune booster.

Orange is known to insulate the body against germs. Not only that, orange essential oil stimulates the lymphatic system. What does that mean? Well, if you have been suffering through a killer cold, it means that your nose that had previously been running like a faucet, will finally get some much-needed relief!

Orange essential oil also works as preventative medicine helping to boost your immune system enough so that you don't get that said cold in the first place! In order to create your own batch of orange essential oil to use in aromatherapy just take 3 drops of orange oil, add in one drop of jasmine oil and add to a good carrier oil such as almond, place in an incense burner or diffuser and breathe in the air!

If you are in need of a serious immune booster, give this one a try. You are going to love it! And the same could be said for all of the immune boosting oils presented here in this final chapter of this book.

Conclusion: Just a Matter of Finding the Right Ingredients

Essential oils are powerful champions of health. Several years of experience are not necessary for you to figure this out. All it really takes is a few whiffs of a strong batch of essential oil recipes and you will quickly become a believer for yourself. The natural world has indeed endowed humanity with a priceless treasure when it comes to essential oils.

In the past people believed that there was something almost sacred and supernatural in the way that these essential oils managed to get people delivered from their maladies.

But looking back at this ancient practice through a more modern lens we realize that it isn't magic that is causing this revitalization, it's a strong physiological response to just the right motivating chemicals.

This doesn't at all take away from the life changing abilities of these oils, it just helps us to better understand the ways in which they work so that we can utilize them to their fullest potential. That is the main drive and purpose of this entire book.

And I sincerely hope that the recipes presented here will be able to aid you in recovering from whatever may be troubling you. Because in the end its all just a matter of finding the right ingredients.

Thank you for reading and good luck!